# Air Fryer Cookbook 2021

Healthy and Easy Recipes for Beginners.

Tips & Tricks to Fry, Grill, Roast, and

Bake.

Your Everyday Air Fryer Book.

Amanda  Grace

# TABLE OF CONTENTS

# INTRODUCTION

## What Is It?

Air Fryer is a kitchen appliance that offers you the convenience of the countertop convection oven, air fryer, toaster, slow cooker, dehydrator, and pizza oven all at once. It can roast food for large families and gatherings, dehydrate snacks without preservatives or added sugar, and air fry French fries without oil.

It uses 360°quick-cook technology with five heating elements thus cooking your meals evenly and quickly. Don't forget the display with 12 preset cooking settings including bake, air fry, Dehydrate, rotisserie, warm, reheat, toast, and roast, bagel, broil, pizza, and slow cook. It also has a sleek stainless-steel construction that highly complements your kitchen and other appliances in it.

## Know About Its Buttons and Functions

Now let's have a look at Air Fryer preset functions.

## Air fry

This is a fast healthy convection cooking method that can be used to replace the messy deep-frying cooking method. Air frying is great for breaded foods with little or no oil. It cooks food by heating from the side heating element and uses the crisper tray in position 4.

## Toast

It is used to crisp and brown bread on both sides. It's a great choice for English muffins or loaves of bread. It heats food with both top and bottom heating elements and uses the pizza rack in position 2.

## Bagel

It's used to crisp and brown thick bread on both sides. It's also good at toasting bagels, frozen waffles, and rolls. It heats food with both the top and bottom heating elements and uses the pizza rack in position 2.

## Pizza

The function is perfect for cooking homemade pizza. It melts the cheese on the top while crisping the dough. It heats food with the top and bottom heating elements and uses the pizza rack in position 5.

## Bake

This function is perfect for pastries such as cakes, cookies, pies and others. It cooks the food using the top and bottom elements and the pizza rack in position 5. You can also use the baking tray if you like.

## Broil

The broiling function is good for searing a piece of meat, melting cheese on food, and cooks open-face sandwiches. It uses the top heating element and uses the baking pan or the pizza rack in position 1 or 2.

## Rotisserie

It's perfect for cooking a whole chicken. The function cooks the food evenly and keeps the food crispy on the outside while juicy on the inside. It uses the top and bottom heating elements and the pizza rack in potion 6.

## Slow cook

The function cooks food at low temperatures for longer times. It's perfect for tough meat cuts. It heats food with the top and bottom elements and uses the pizza rack in position 6.

## Roast

Perfect for large pieces of poultry and other meat. The function cooks food using the top and bottom elements and uses the pizza rack in position 5.

## Dehydrate

Dehydration is perfect for drying fruits, meats, and vegetables. It cooks food in a convection way on low heat. It heats food using the top heating element and uses the crisper tray in positions 1, 4, and 5.

## Reheat

The function is used to heat already prepared meals without overcooking them. It uses the top and bottom heating elements to reheat food with the pizza rack in position 5.

## Warm

The warm setting holds up food at a safe warm temperature for a certain period of time. It warms food using the top and bottom heating elements and uses the crisper tray, the pizza rack, or the baking pan in potion 5.

## It Also Comes with Some Knobs and Buttons;

### Temperature/ darkness control knob

The knob allows you to adjust the preset temperature and to control the amount of light during toast or bagel.

### Time/ slices control knob

The knob allows you to adjust the preset time and also to select the number of slices you want to toast or bagel.

### Program selection knob

Allows you to check the preset choices and select one.

### Air fry button

Push the button to air fry food or activate the air frying fan for other preset functions.

## Light button

Used to light up the interior of the appliance while cooking.

## Temperature button

It has °F and °C temperature units and you can choose your preferred method to mature the cooking temperature.

## Cancel button

Used to the current cooking process and can power off the unit by pressing it for long. (3 seconds)

## Start/ pause button

Starts or pauses the cooking process.

# The Work Mechanism

The Air Fryer uses the 360° quick-cook heat technology. This means that you can cook a whole chicken with half an hour less the time you would cook it in a convection oven. The good news is the Air Fryer heats up very fast so there's no need to wait until it preheats. You can even cook frozen food directly by just adding a few minutes to the actual cooking time and the food will come out perfectly.

This amazing kitchen appliance comes with a number of accessories. Let's talk how they work.

## The pizza racks

Insert the drip tray at the very bottom of the appliance then use the markings on the door to place the pizza rack on the ideal position or as recommended on the recipe.

## The baking trays

Insert the drip tray at the very bottom of the appliance then use the markings on the door to place the pizza rack as recommended on the recipe. Place the baking pan on the pizza rack and then place the food on the baking tray.

**The crisper tray**

Insert the drip tray at the very bottom of the appliance then use the markings on the door to place the crisper tray as recommended on the recipe. Place the food on the crisp tray.

**The rotisserie spit**

Insert the drip tray at the very bottom of the appliance. Remove the forks, and force the rotisserie spit through the food center lengthwise. Now slide the forks on both sides and tighten them with the set screws. Now insert the rotisserie spit into the rotisserie connections in the appliance. Your food is now ready to be cooked as recommended in the recipe.

# Pros of Using It

1. Using 360°quick-cook turbo heat technology makes it super-fast compared to other cooking appliances thus saving on energy and time.
2. Its versatile, and can act as a toaster, dehydrator, rotisserie, slow cooker among others.
3. Easy to clean and maintain. The accessories are dishwasher safe but it is advisable to hand wash them.
4. Very easy to use. With the preset functions, one can easily cook any type of food using the unit.

5. Cooking without oil thus cutting on the intake of calories from oils and fat.

# BREAKFAST

## Turkey Morning Patties

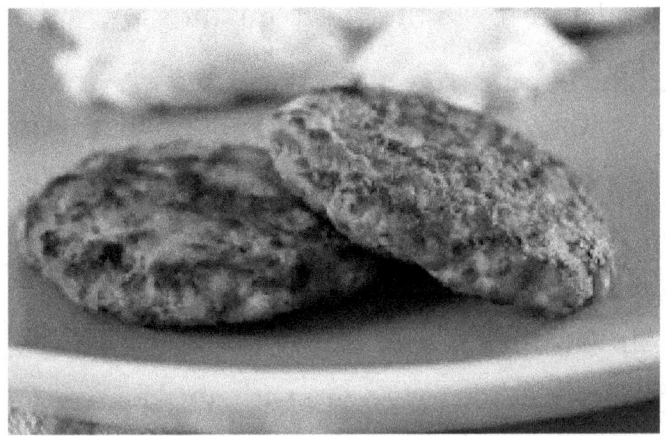

Preparation Time: 10 Minutes

Cooking Time: 13 Minutes

Servings: 8

**Ingredients:**

- 2 tsp fennel seeds
- 1 lb. pork mince
- 2 tsp dry rubbed sage
- 1 lb. turkey mince
- 2 tsp garlic powder
- 1 tsp paprika

- 1 tsp sea salt
- 1 tsp dried thyme

**Directions:**

1. In a mixing bowl, add turkey and pork then mix them together.
2. Mix sage, fennel, paprika, salt, thyme, and garlic powder in a small bowl.
3. Drizzle this mixture over the meat mixture and mix well.
4. Take 2 tbsp of this mixture at a time and roll it into thick patties.
5. Place half of the patties in the Basket 1, and the other half in basket 2 then spray them all with cooking oil.
6. Return the Air Fryer Baskets to the Air Fryer.
7. Select the Air Fryer mode for Zone 1 with 390 degrees F temperature and 13 minutes cooking time.
8. Press the MATCH COOK button to copy the settings for Zone 2.
9. Initiate cooking by pressing the START/PAUSE BUTTON.
10. Flip the patties in the baskets once cooked halfway through.
11. Serve warm and fresh.

**Nutrition:** Calories 184 Total Fat 7.9 g Saturated Fat 1.4 g Cholesterol 36 mg Sodium 704 mg Total Carbs 6 g Fiber 3.6 g Sugar 5.5 g Protein 17.9 g

# Potato Hash Browns

Preparation Time: 10 Minutes

Cooking Time: 13 Minutes

Servings: 6

## Ingredients:

- 3 russet potatoes
- ¼ cup chopped green peppers
- ¼ cup chopped red peppers
- ¼ cup chopped onions
- 2 garlic cloves chopped
- 1 tsp paprika
- Salt and black pepper, to taste
- 2 tsp olive oil

## Directions:

1. Peel and grate all the potatoes with the help of a cheese grater.
2. Add potato shreds to a bowl filled with cold water and leave it soaked for 25 minutes.
3. Drain the water and place the potato shreds in a plate lined with a paper towel.
4. Transfer the shreds to a dry bowl and add olive oil, paprika, garlic, and black pepper.

5.  Make four flat patties out of the potato mixture and place two into each of the Air fryer baskets.

6.  Return the Air Fryer Baskets to the Air Fryer.

7.  Select the Air Fryer mode for Zone 1 with 390 degrees F temperature and 13 minutes cooking time.

8.  Press the MATCH COOK button to copy the settings for Zone 2.

9.  Initiate cooking by pressing the START/PAUSE BUTTON.

10. Flip the potato hash browns once cooked halfway through, then resume cooking.

11. Once done, serve warm.

**Nutrition:** Calories 134 Total Fat 4.7 g Saturated Fat 0.6 g Cholesterol 124mg Sodium 1 mg Total Carbs 54.1 g Fiber 7 g Sugar 3.3 g Protein 6.2 g

# Air Fried Breakfast Sausage

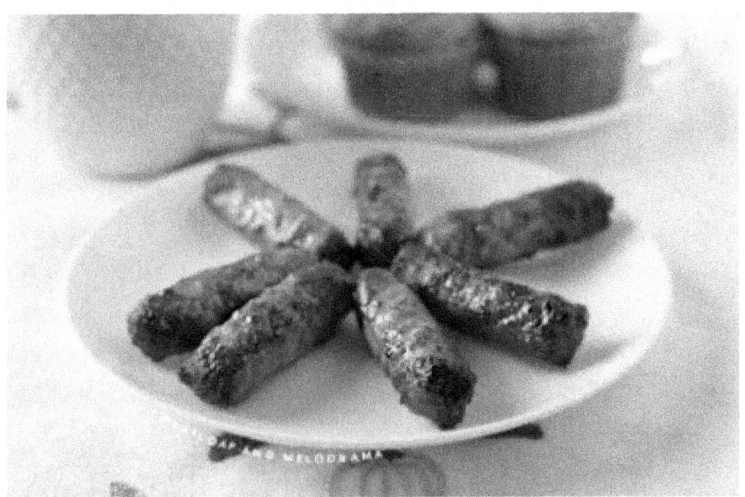

Preparation Time: 10 Minutes

Cooking Time: 13 Minutes

Servings: 4

**Ingredients:**

- 4 sausage links, raw and uncooked

**Directions:**

1. Divide the sausages in the two Air fryer baskets.
2. Return the Air Fryer Baskets to the Air Fryer.
3. Select the Air Fryer mode for Zone 1 with 390 degrees F temperature and 13 minutes cooking time.
4. Press the MATCH COOK button to copy the settings for Zone 2.
5. Initiate cooking by pressing the START/PAUSE BUTTON.
6. Serve warm and fresh.

**Nutrition:** Calories 187 Total Fat 6 g Saturated Fat 9.9 g Cholesterol 41 mg  Sodium 154 mg Total Carbs 7.4 g Fiber 2.9 g Sugar 15.3 g Protein 24.6 g

# Egg Pepper Cups

Preparation Time: 10 Minutes

Cooking Time: 12 Minutes

Servings: 4

**Ingredients:**

- 2 bell pepper, halved, seeds removed
- 8 eggs
- 1 tsp olive oil
- 1 pinch salt and black pepper
- 1 pinch sriracha flakes

**Directions:**

1. Slice the bell peppers in half, lengthwise and remove their seeds and the inner portion to get cup-like shape.
2. Rub olive oil on the edges of the bell peppers.
3. Place them in the two Air Fryer Baskets with their cut side up and crack two eggs in each half of bell pepper.
4. Drizzle salt, black pepper, and sriracha flakes on top of the eggs.
5. Return the Air Fryer Baskets to the Air Fryer.
6. Select the Air Fryer mode for Zone 1 with 390 degrees F temperature and 18 minutes cooking time.
7. Press the MATCH COOK button to copy the settings for Zone 2.

8. Initiate cooking by pressing the START/PAUSE BUTTON.

9. Serve warm and fresh.

**Nutrition:** Calories 212 Total Fat 11.8 g Saturated Fat 2.2 g Cholesterol 23mg Sodium 321 mg Total Carbs 14.6 g Dietary Fiber 4.4 g Sugar 8 g Protein 17.3 g

# Crispy Breakfast Bacon

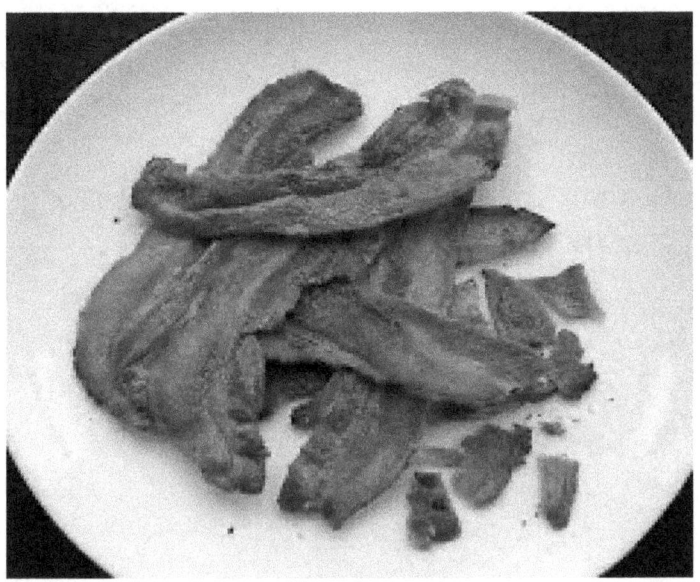

Preparation Time: 10 Minutes

Cooking Time: 14 Minutes

Servings: 6

**Ingredients:**

- ½ lb. of bacon slices

**Directions:**

1. Spread half of the bacon slices in each of the Air Fryer baskets evenly in a single layer.

2. Return the Air Fryer Baskets to the Air Fryer.

3. Select the Air Fryer mode for Zone 1 with 390 degrees F temperature and 14 minutes cooking time.

4. Press the MATCH COOK button to copy the settings for Zone 2.

5. Initiate cooking by pressing the START/PAUSE BUTTON.

6. Flip the crispy bacon once cooked halfway through, then resume cooking.

7. Serve.

**Nutrition:** Calories 142 Total Fat 24.8 g Saturated Fat 12.4 g Cholesterol 3 mg Sodium 132 mg Total Carbs 0.8 g Dietary Fiber 3.9 g Sugar 2.5 g Protein 18.9 g

# Egg Bacon Balls

Preparation Time: 10 Minutes

Cooking Time: 14 Minutes

Servings: 6

**Ingredients:**

- 1 tbsp butter
- 2 eggs, beaten
- ¼ tsp pepper
- 1 can (10.2 oz) Pillsbury Buttermilk biscuits
- 2 oz cheddar cheese, diced into ten cubes
- Cooking spray
- Egg Wash
- 1 egg
- 1 tbsp water

**Directions:**

1. Place a suitable non-stick skillet over medium-high heat and cook the bacon until crispy, then place it in a plate lined with a paper towel.
2. Melt butter in the same skillet over medium heat. Beat eggs with pepper in a bowl and pour them in the skillet.
3. Stir cook for 5 minutes then remove it from the heat.
4. Add bacon and mix well.

5. Divide the dough into 5 biscuits and slice each into 2 layers.

6. Press each biscuit into 4 inches round.

7. Add a tbsp of egg mixture at the center of each round and top it with a piece of cheese.

8. Carefully fold the biscuit dough around the filling and pinch the edges to seal.

9. Whisk egg with water in a small bowl and brush the egg wash over the biscuits.

10. Place the half of the biscuit bombs in each of the Air Fryer Baskets and spray them with cooking oil.

11. Return the Air Fryer Baskets to the Air Fryer.

12. Select the Air Fryer mode for Zone 1 with 375 degrees F temperature and 14 minutes cooking time.

13. Press the MATCH COOK button to copy the settings for Zone 2.

14. Initiate cooking by pressing the START/PAUSE BUTTON.

15. Flip the egg bombs when cooked halfway through, then resume cooking.

16. Serve warm.

**Nutrition:** Calories 331 Total Fat 2.5 g Saturated Fat 0.5 g Cholesterol 35 mg Sodium 595 mg Total Carbs 29 g Fiber 12.2 g Sugar 12.5 g Protein 18.7g

# Crispy Egg Rolls

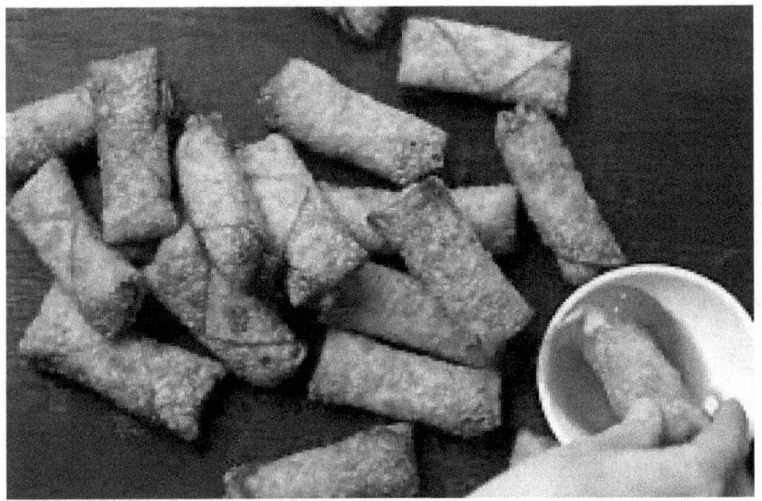

Preparation Time: 10 Minutes

Cooking Time: 13 Minutes

Servings: 6

**Ingredients:**

- 2 eggs
- 2 tbsp milk
- Salt, to taste
- Black pepper, to taste
- 1/2 cup shredded cheddar cheese
- 2 sausage patties
- 6 egg roll wrappers
- 1 tbsp olive oil

- 1 cup of water

**Directions:**

1. Grease a small skillet with some olive oil and place it over medium heat.
2. Add sausage patties and cook them until brown.
3. Chop the cooked patties into small pieces. Beat eggs with salt, black pepper, and milk in a mixing bowl.
4. Grease the same skillet with 1 tsp olive oil and pour the egg mixture into it.
5. Stir cook to make scrambled eggs.
6. Add sausage, mix well and remove the skillet from the heat.
7. Spread an egg roll wrapper on the working surface in a diamond shape position.
8. Add a tbsp of cheese at the bottom third of the roll wrapper.
9. Top the cheese with egg mixture and wet the edges of the wrapper with water.
10. Fold the two corners of the wrapper and roll it then seal the edges.
11. Repeat the same steps and divide the rolls in the two Air Fryer Baskets.
12. Return the Air Fryer Baskets to the Air Fryer.
13. Select the Air Fryer mode for Zone 1 with 375 degrees F temperature and 13 minutes cooking time.

14. Press the MATCH COOK button to copy the settings for Zone 2.

15. Initiate cooking by pressing the START/PAUSE BUTTON.

16. Flip the rolls after 8 minutes and continue cooking for another 5 minutes.

17. Serve warm and fresh.

**Nutrition:** Calories 322 Total Fat 11.8 g Saturated Fat 2.2 g Cholesterol 56 mg  Sodium 321 mg Total Carbs 14.6 g Dietary Fiber 4.4 g Sugar 8 g Protein 17.3 g

# Spinach Egg Cups

Preparation Time: 10 Minutes

Cooking Time: 13 Minutes

Servings: 4

**Ingredients:**

- 4 tbsp milk
- 4 tbsp frozen spinach, thawed
- 4 large egg
- 8 tsp grated cheese
- Salt, to taste
- Black pepper, to taste
- Cooking Spray

**Directions:**

1. Grease four small sized ramekin with cooking spray.
2. Add egg, cheese, spinach, and milk to a bowl and beat well.
3. Divide the mixture into the four small ramekins and top them with salt and black pepper.
4. Place the two ramekins in each of the two Air Fryer Baskets.
5. Return the Air Fryer Baskets to the Air Fryer.
6. Select the Air Fryer mode for Zone 1 with 390 degrees F temperature and 13 minutes cooking time.

7. Press the MATCH COOK button to copy the settings for Zone 2.

8. Initiate cooking by pressing the START/PAUSE BUTTON.

9. Serve warm.

**Nutrition:** Calories 197 Total Fat 15.4 g Saturated Fat 4.2 g Cholesterol 168 mg  Sodium 203 mg Total Carbs 8.5 g Sugar 1.1 g Fiber 4 g Protein 17.9 g

# French Toast Sticks

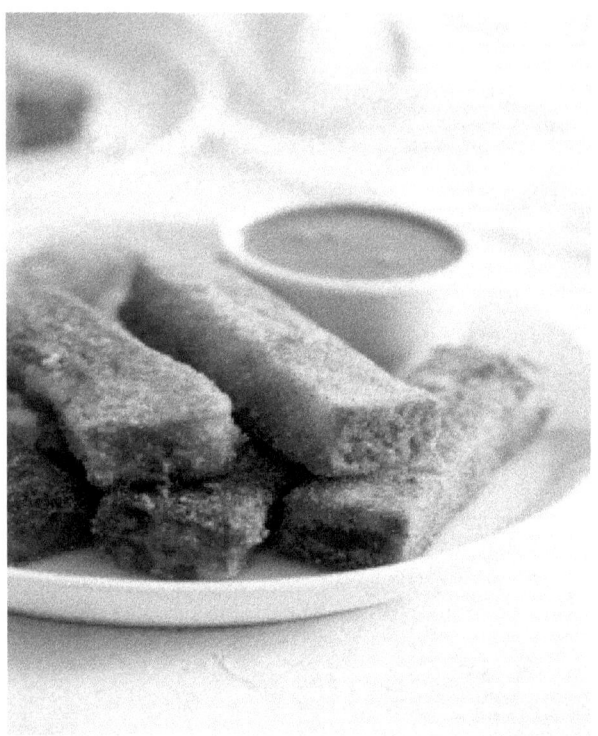

Preparation Time: 10 Minutes

Cooking Time: 8 Minutes

Servings: 2

**Ingredients:**

- 4 pieces of bread
- 2 tbsp butter
- 2 eggs, beaten
- 1 pinch salt

- 1 pinch cinnamon ground
- 1 pinch nutmeg ground
- 1 pinch ground clove
- 1 tsp icing sugar

**Directions:**

1. Add two eggs to a mixing bowl and stir cinnamon, nutmeg, ground cloves, and salt, then whisk well.
2. Spread butter on both sides of the bread slices and cut them into thick strips.
3. Dip the breadsticks in the egg mixture and place them in the two Air Fryer baskets.
4. Return the Air Fryer Baskets to the Air Fryer.
5. Select the Air Fryer mode for Zone 1 with 390 degrees F temperature and 8 minutes cooking time.
6. Press the MATCH COOK button to copy the settings for Zone 2.
7. Initiate cooking by pressing the START/PAUSE BUTTON.
8. Flip the French toast sticks when cooked halfway through.
9. Serve.

**Nutrition:** Calories 391 Total Fat 2.8 g Saturated Fat 0.6 g Cholesterol 330 mg  Sodium 62 mg Total Carbs 36.5 g Fiber 9.2 g Sugar 4.5 g  Protein 6.6

# Tasty Coconut Almond Donuts

Preparation Time: 5 Minutes

Cooking Time: 25 Minutes

Servings: 4

**Ingredients:**

- 2 tablespoons almond flour
- 1-tablespoon coconut flour
- ½ tablespoon psyllium husk
- ½ teaspoon xanthan gum
- ½ cup unsweetened almond milk
- 2 tablespoons coconut oil
- A pinch of salt
- 2 eggs
- 1-tablespoon extra-virgin olive oil

**Directions:**

1. Combine the almond flour with coconut flour then add psyllium husk, xanthan gum, and salt. Mix well.
2. Add egg to the flour mixture then pour coconut oil and almond milk to them mixture.
3. Knead the mixture until it becomes dough then divide the dough into 8.
4. Shape each part of the dough into a donut form then arrange them on a flat surface.

5. Install the crisper plate into the basket of your Ninja Foodi then preheat the Ninja Foodi for 3 minutes.
6. Select the "Air Fry" menu then set the time to 5 minutes.
7. Arrange the donut in the Ninja Foodi's basket then spray olive oil over them.
8. Press the "Start/Stop" button to begin then fry the donuts.
9. Once then Ninja Foodi beeps and the donuts are done, remove them from the Ninja Foodi, and arrange them on a serving dish. Repeat with the remaining donuts.
10. Once it is done, arrange the donuts on a serving dish and serve.
11. Enjoy it!

**Nutrition:** 157 Calories, 13.7g Fats, 7.6g Net Carbs, 3.6g Protein

# LUNCH

## Parmesan Chicken Meatballs

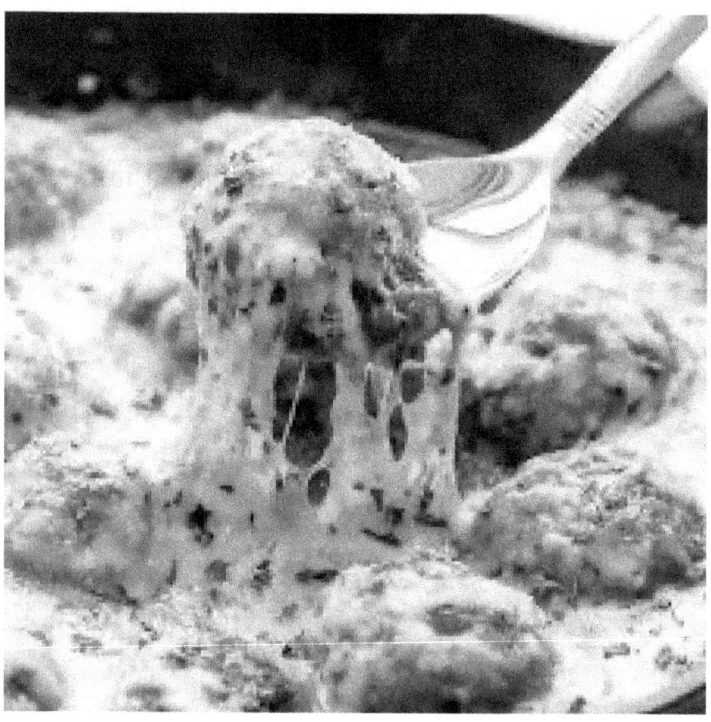

Preparation Time: 10 minutes

Cooking Time: 12 Minutes

Servings: 4

**Ingredients:**

- 1-lb. ground chicken
- 1 large egg, beaten

- ½ cup Parmesan cheese, grated
- ½ cup pork rinds, ground
- 1 teaspoon garlic powder
- 1 teaspoon paprika
- 1 teaspoon kosher salt
- ½ teaspoon pepper
- Crust:
- ½ cup pork rinds, ground

## Directions:

1. Toss all the meatball Ingredients: in a bowl and mix well.
2. Make small meatballs out this mixture and roll them in the pork rinds.
3. Place the coated meatballs in the air fryer basket.
4. Press "Power Button" of Air Fry Oven and turn the dial to select the "Bake" mode.
5. Press the Time button and again turn the dial to set the cooking time to 12 minutes.
6. Now push the Temp button and rotate the dial to set the temperature at 400 degrees F.
7. Once preheated, place the air fryer basket inside and close its lid.
8. Serve warm.

**Nutrition:** Calories 529 Total Fat 17 g Saturated Fat 3 g Cholesterol 65 mg Sodium 391 mg Total Carbs 55 g
Fiber 6 g Sugar 8 g Protein 41g

# Creamy Green Beans and Tomatoes

Preparation Time: 10 minutes

Cooking Time: 20 Minutes

Servings: 4

**Ingredients:**

- 1-pound green beans, trimmed and halved
- ½ pound cherry tomatoes, halved
- 2 tablespoons olive oil
- 1 teaspoon oregano, dried
- 1 teaspoon basil, dried
- Salt and black pepper to the taste
- 1 cup heavy cream
- ½ tablespoon cilantro, chopped

**Directions:**

1. In your air fryer's pan, combine the green beans with the tomatoes and the other Ingredients: toss and cook at 360 degrees F for 20 minutes.
2. Divide the mix between plates and serve.

**Nutrition:** Calories 174fat 5 fiber 7 carbs 11 protein 4

# Carrot and Beef Cocktail Balls

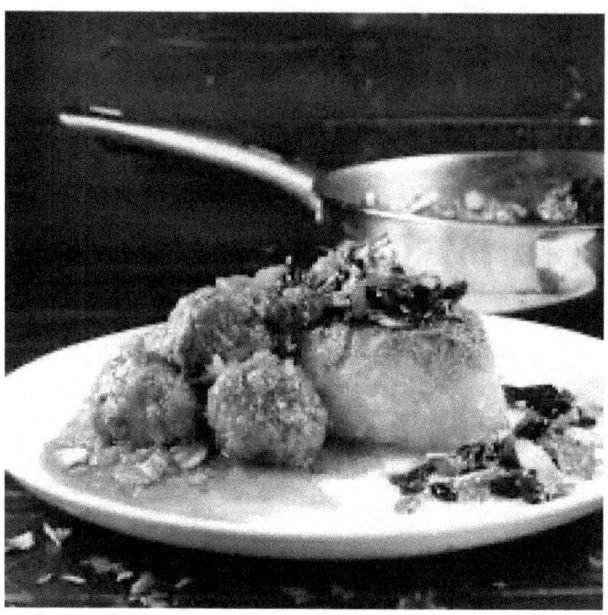

Preparation Time: 10 minutes

Cooking Time: 20 Minutes

Servings: 10

**Ingredients:**

- 1-pound ground beef
- 2 carrots
- 1 red onion, peeled and chopped
- 2 cloves garlic
- 1/2 teaspoon dried rosemary, crushed
- 1/2 teaspoon dried basil
- 1 teaspoon dried oregano

- 1 egg
- 3/4 cup breadcrumbs
- 1/2 teaspoon salt
- 1/2 teaspoon black pepper, or to taste
- 1 cup plain flour

**Directions:**

1. Preparing the ingredients. Place ground beef in a large bowl.
2. In a food processor, pulse the carrot, onion and garlic; transfer the vegetable mixture to a large-sized bowl.
3. Then, add the rosemary, basil, oregano, egg, breadcrumbs, salt, and black pepper.
4. Shape the mixture into even balls; refrigerate for about 30 minutes.
5. Roll the balls into the flour.
6. Air frying. Close air fryer lid.
7. Then, air-fry the balls at 350 degrees f for about 20 minutes, turning occasionally; work with batches. Serve with toothpicks.

**Nutrition:** Calories 284 Total fat 7.9 g Saturated fat 1.4 g Cholesterol 36 mg Sodium 704 mg Total carbs 46 g
Fiber 3.6 g Sugar 5.5 g Protein 17.9 g

# Lamb Gyro

Preparation Time: 10 minutes

Cooking Time: 25 Minutes

Servings: 4

**Ingredients:**

- 1 pound ground lamb
- ¼ red onion, minced
- ¼ cup mint, minced
- ¼ cup parsley, minced
- 2 cloves garlic, minced
- ½ teaspoon salt
- ⅛ teaspoon rosemary
- ½ teaspoon black pepper
- 4 slices pita bread
- ¾ cup hummus
- 1 cup romaine lettuce, shredded
- ½ onion sliced
- 1 Roma tomato, diced
- ½ cucumber, skinned and thinly sliced
- 12 mint leaves, minced
- Tzatziki sauce, to taste

**Directions:**

1. Mix ground lamb, red onion, mint, parsley, garlic, salt, rosemary, and black pepper until fully incorporated.

2. Select the Broil function on the COSORI Air Fryer Toaster Oven, set time to 25 minutes and temperature to 450°F, then press Start/Cancel to preheat.

3. Line the food tray with parchment paper and place ground lamb on top, shaping it into a patty 1-inch-thick and 6 inches in diameter.

4. Insert the food tray at top position in the preheated air fryer toaster oven, then press Start/Cancel.

5. Remove when done and cut into thin slices.

6. Assemble each gyro starting with pita bread, then hummus, lamb meat, lettuce, onion, tomato, cucumber, and mint leaves, then drizzle with tzatziki.

7. Serve immediately.

**Nutrition:** Calories: 409 kcal Total Fat: 14.6 g Saturated Fat: 0 g Cholesterol: 0 mg Sodium: 0 mg Total Carbs: 29.9 g Fiber: 0 g Sugar: 0 g Protein: 39.4 g

# Air Fryer Fish

Preparation Time: 10 minutes

Cooking Time: 17 Minutes

Servings: 4

**Ingredients:**

- 4-6 Whiting Fish fillets cut in half
- Oil to mist
- Fish Seasoning
- ¾ cup very fine cornmeal
- ¼ cup flour
- 2 tsp old bay
- 1 ½ tsp salt
- 1 tsp paprika
- ½ tsp garlic powder
- ½ tsp black pepper

**Directions:**

1. Put the Ingredients: for fish seasoning in a Ziplock bag and shake it well. Set aside.
2. Rinse and pat dry the fish fillets with paper towels. Make sure that they still are damp.
3. Place the fish fillets in a Ziplock bag and shake until they are completely covered with seasoning.

4. Place the fillets on a baking rack to let any excess flour to fall off.

5. Grease the bottom of the Instant Pot Duo Crisp Air Fryer basket tray and place the fillets on the tray. Close the lid, select the Air Fry option and cook filets on 400°F for 10 minutes.

6. Open the Air Fryer lid and spray the fish with oil on the side facing up before flipping it over, ensure that the fish is fully coated. Flip and cook another side of the fish for 7 minutes. Remove the fish and serve.

**Nutrition:** Calories 193 Total Fat 1g Total Carbs 27g Protein 19g

# Cheese-stuffed Meatballs

Preparation Time: 10 minutes

Cooking Time: 10 Minutes

Servings: 4

**Ingredients:**

- ⅓ cup soft bread crumbs
- 3 tablespoons milk
- 1 tablespoon ketchup
- 1 egg
- ½ teaspoon dried marjoram
- Pinch salt
- Freshly ground black pepper
- 1-pound 95 percent lean ground beef
- 20 ½-inch cubes of cheese
- Olive oil for misting

**Directions:**

1. Preparing the ingredients. In a large bowl, combine the bread crumbs, milk, ketchup, egg, marjoram, salt, and pepper, and mix well. Add the ground beef and mix gently but thoroughly with your hands. Form the mixture into 20 meatballs. Shape each meatball around a cheese cube. Mist the meatballs with olive oil and put into the instant crisp air fryer basket.

2. Air frying. Close air fryer lid. Bake for 10 to 13 minutes or until the meatballs register 165°f on a meat thermometer.

**Nutrition:** Calories: 393 Fat: 17g Protein:50g Fiber:0g

# Sweet Potato and Parsnip Spiralized Latkes

Preparation Time: 10 minutes

Cooking Time: 20 Minutes

Servings: 12

**Ingredients:**

- 1 medium sweet potato
- 1 large parsnip
- 4 cups water
- 1 egg + 1 egg white
- 2 scallions
- 1/2 teaspoon garlic powder
- 1/2 teaspoon sea salt
- 1/2 teaspoon ground pepper

**Directions:**

1. Start by spiralizing the sweet potato and parsnip and chopping the scallions, reserving only the green parts.
2. Preheat toaster oven to 425°F.
3. Bring 4 cups of water to a boil. Place all of your noodles in a colander and pour the boiling water over the top, draining well.

4. Let the noodles cool, then grab handfuls and place them in a paper towel; squeeze to remove as much liquid as possible.

5. In a large bowl, beat egg and egg white together. Add noodles, scallions, garlic powder, salt, and pepper, mix well.

6. Prepare a baking sheet; scoop out 1/4 cup of mixture at a time and place on sheet.

7. Slightly press down each scoop with your hands, then bake for 20 minutes, flipping halfway through.

**Nutrition:** Calories: 24 Sodium: 91 mg Dietary Fiber: 1.0 g Total Fat: 0.4 g Total Carbs: 4.3 g Protein: 0.9 g.

# Chicken Breasts with Chimichurri

Preparation Time: 10 minutes

Cooking Time: 35 Minutes

Servings: 1

**Ingredients:**

- 1 chicken breast, bone-in, skin-on
- Chimichurri
- ½ bunch fresh cilantro
- 1/4 bunch fresh parsley
- ½ shallot, peeled, cut in quarters
- ½ tablespoon paprika ground
- ½ tablespoon chili powder
- ½ tablespoon fennel ground
- ½ teaspoon black pepper, ground
- ½ teaspoon onion powder
- 1 teaspoon salt
- ½ teaspoon garlic powder
- ½ teaspoon cumin ground
- ½ tablespoon canola oil
- Chimichurri
- 2 tablespoons olive oil
- 4 garlic cloves, peeled

- Zest and juice of 1 lemon
- 1 teaspoon kosher salt

**Directions:**

1. Preheat the Air fryer to 300-degree F and grease an Air fryer basket.
2. Combine all the spices in a suitable bowl and season the chicken with it.
3. Sprinkle with canola oil and arrange the chicken in the Air fryer basket.
4. Cook for about 35 minutes and dish out in a platter.
5. Put all the ingredients in the blender and blend until smooth.
6. Serve the chicken with chimichurri sauce.

**Nutrition:** Calories: 140 Fats: 7.9g Carbohydrates: 1.8g Sugar: 7.1g Proteins: 7.2g Sodium: 581mg

# Turkey and Almonds

Preparation Time: 10 minutes

Cooking Time: 10 Minutes

Servings: 2

**Ingredients:**

- 1 big turkey breast, skinless; boneless and halved
- 2 shallots; chopped
- 1/3 cup almonds; chopped
- 1 tbsp. sweet paprika
- 2 tbsp. olive oil
- Salt and black pepper to taste.

**Directions:**

1. In a pan that fits the air fryer, combine the turkey with all the other ingredients, toss.
2. Put the pan in the machine and cook at 370°F for 25 minutes
3. Divide everything between plates and serve.

**Nutrition:** Calories: 274 Fat: 12g Fiber: 3g Carbs: 5g Protein: 14g

# Balsamic Roasted Chicken

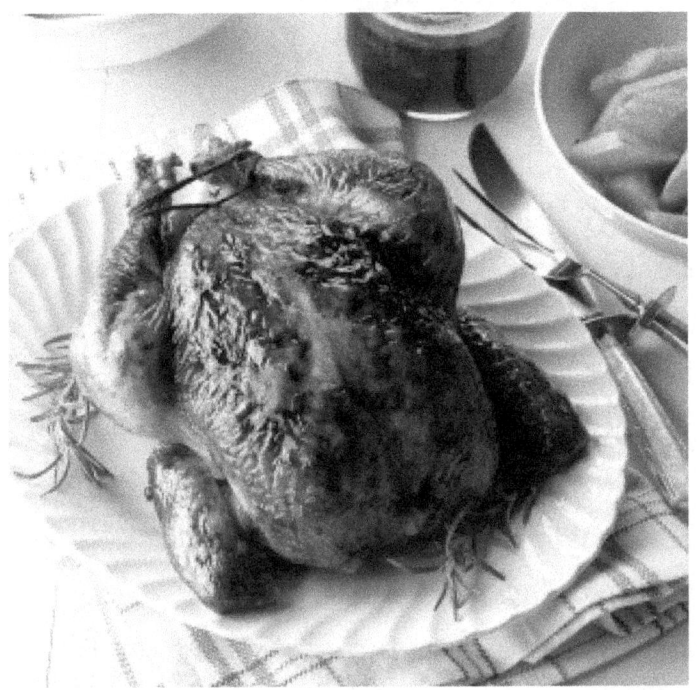

Preparation Time: 10 minutes

Cooking Time: 1 hour

Servings: 4

**Ingredients:**

- 1/2 cup balsamic vinegar
- 1/4 cup Dijon mustard
- 1/3 cup olive oil
- Juice and zest from 1 lemon
- 3 minced garlic cloves

- 1 teaspoon salt
- 1 teaspoon pepper
- 4 bone-in, skin-on chicken thighs
- 4 bone-in, skin-on chicken drumsticks
- 1 tablespoon chopped parsley

**Directions:**

1. Mix vinegar, lemon juice, mustard, olive oil, garlic, salt, and pepper in a bowl, then pour into a sauce pan.
2. Roll chicken pieces in the pan, then cover and marinate for at least 2 hours, but up to 24 hours.
3. Preheat the toaster oven to 400°F and place the chicken on a fresh baking sheet, reserving the marinade for later.
4. Roast the chicken for 50 minutes.
5. Remove the chicken and cover it with foil to keep it warm. Place the marinade in the toaster oven for about 5 minutes until it simmers down and begins to thicken.
6. Pour marinade over chicken and sprinkle with parsley and lemon zest.

**Nutrition:** Calories: 1537 Sodium: 1383 mg Dietary Fiber: 0.8 g Total Fat: 70.5 g Total Carbs: 2.4 g Protein: 210.4 g.

# DINNER

## Lemony-Honey Roasted Radishes

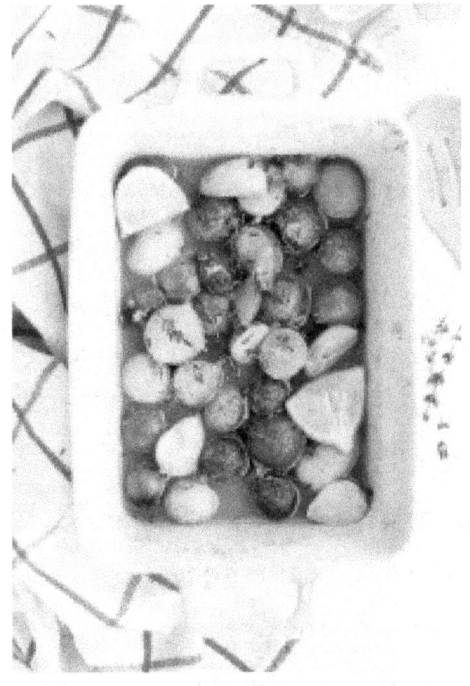

Preparation time: 10 minutes

Cooking time: 17 minutes

Servings: 4

## Ingredients

- 1-pound (454 g) radishes, with green leaves attached
- 1 tablespoon extra-virgin olive oil
- 1 tablespoon white balsamic vinegar
- 1 preserved lemon, flesh discarded, rind cut into shreds, plus 2 tablespoons brine from the jar, plus more if needed
- 1 tablespoon unsalted butter
- Sea salt flakes and freshly ground black pepper, to taste
- 1½ tablespoons clear honey
- Leaves from 6 mint sprigs, torn

## Directions

1. Wash the radishes well and remove their leaves.
2. Halve the radishes lengthwise. Put them in a baking pan with the olive oil, white balsamic, half the preserved lemon brine, and all the butter. Season.
3. Select Bake. Set temperature to 400°F (205°C) and set time to 17 minutes. Select Start to begin preheating.
4. Once preheated, slide the pan into the oven.
5. After 7 minutes, add the remaining tablespoon of brine and the honey. Shake the pan around and return to the oven for a final 10 minutes.
6. Transfer to a warmed serving dish and mix in the reserved radish leaves; they will wilt in the heat. Stir in the shredded preserved lemon rind and taste for seasoning. Scatter on the mint leaves and serve.

**Nutrition:** Calories 79 Carbs 7 g Protein 5 g Fat 3 g

# Stuffed Peppers with Cheese and Basil

Preparation time: 10 minutes

Cooking time: 40 minutes

Servings: 6

## Ingredients

- 6 medium bell peppers
- A little extra-virgin olive oil
- 5½ ounces (156 g) ricotta (fresh rather than ultra-pasteurized, if possible)
- 10½ ounces (297 g) soft goat cheese
- 1 cup finely grated Parmesan cheese
- Sea salt flakes and freshly ground black pepper, to taste
- 1 cup basil leaves, torn
- 1 large egg
- 1 garlic clove, crushed
- 1 tablespoon toasted pine nuts (optional)

## Directions

1. Halve the peppers, deseed them, brush them with olive oil, and put them into a gratin dish from which they can be served.

2. Drain the ricotta and the goat cheese. Mix together all three cheeses with seasoning, the basil, egg, and garlic, gently mashing. Add the pine nuts if you are using them.

3. Spoon the mixture into the pepper halves and transfer the stuffed peppers to a baking pan.

4. Select Bake. Set temperature to 375°F (190°C) and set time to 40 minutes. Select Start to begin preheating.

5. Once preheated, slide the pan into the oven. When done, the filling should be golden and soufflé and the peppers completely tender when pierced with a sharp knife. If they're not ready, return them to the oven for an extra 5 to 10 minutes, then test again.

**Nutrition:** Calories 79 Carbs 7 g Protein 5 g Fat 3 g

# Oregano Eggplants with Chili Anchovy Sauce

Preparation time: 15 minutes

Cooking time: 40 minutes

Serving: 4

**Ingredients**

- For the Eggplants:
- 4¾ pounds (2.2 kg) globe eggplants
- 4 tablespoons extra-virgin olive oil
- Leaves from 3 oregano sprigs, torn
- Sea salt flakes and freshly ground black pepper, to taste
- Juice of ½ lemon
- Good crusty bread, to serve
- For the Sauce:
- Leaves from 2 rosemary sprigs
- 2 garlic cloves, chopped
- 14 anchovies, drained of oil
- Juice of 1 lemon, or to taste
- 4 tablespoons extra-virgin olive oil
- 1 red Fresno chili, halved, seeded, and chopped, plus more if you want it hotter

**Directions**

1. Halve the eggplants and cut a cross-hatched pattern in the flesh of each one, without cutting all the way through to the skin. Put them on to a rimmed baking sheet—line it with parchment paper or foil if you want and smear the olive oil evenly all over the cut surfaces. Toss in the oregano, too, and salt and pepper. Turn the eggplants over with your hands, making sure the seasoning and some of the herb leaves go into the flesh.

2. Select Bake. Set temperature to 400°F (205°C) and set time to 40 minutes. Select Start to begin preheating.

3. Once preheated, slide the baking sheet into the oven.

4. When done, the eggplants will be completely tender right through and golden. Squeeze the lemon juice over the top.

5. To make the sauce, pound the rosemary and garlic in a mortar, then add the anchovies and crush to a paste. Gradually add the lemon juice and then the olive oil, a little at a time, grinding as you go. You aren't making a mayonnaise—so don't expect this to emulsify, you'll be left with a lumpy "sauce"—but the pounding melds all the elements together. Add the chili and set aside. The longer the sauce sits with the chili, the hotter it will become.

6. Serve the eggplants with the sauce, either on the side or spooned over the top. You need good bread with this, to mop up all the juices.

**Nutrition:** Calories 79 Carbs 7 g Protein 5 g Fat 3 g

# Buttery Eggplant and Tomato with Freekeh

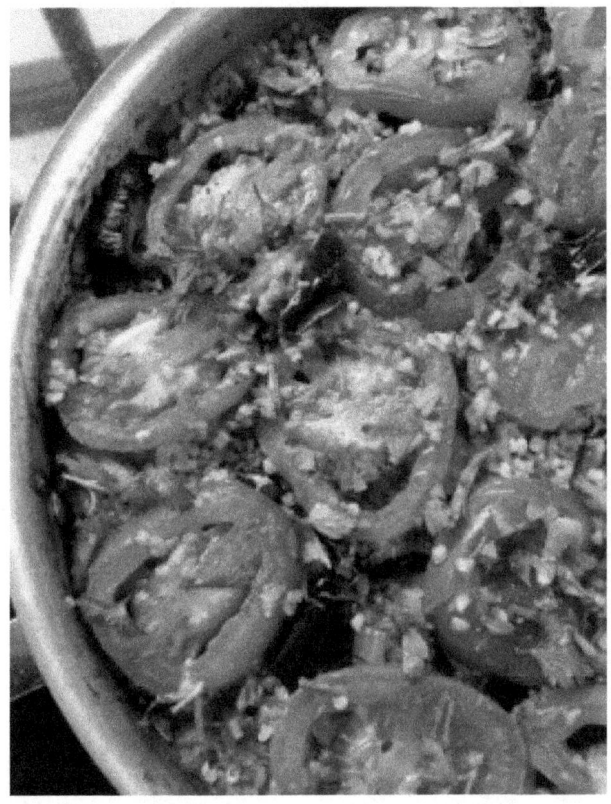

Preparation time: 20 minutes

Cooking time: 30 minutes

Servings: 4

**Ingredients**

- For the Vegetables and Freekeh:
- 2¼ pounds (1 kg) baby eggplants

- 2¼ pounds (1 kg) plum tomatoes
- 7 tablespoons unsalted butter
- 12 garlic cloves, thickly sliced
- Sea salt flakes and freshly ground black pepper, to taste
- A little light brown sugar (optional, only if your tomatoes aren't sweet)
- Scant 2 cups cooked freekeh
- Plain yogurt, to serve
- Good bread, to serve
- For the Koch-Kocha:
- ½ green bell pepper, halved, seeded, and roughly chopped
- 4 cups cilantro leaves
- 1 red Fresno chili and 1 green chili, halved and deseeded
- 1¼-inch fresh ginger, peeled and finely grated
- Juice of 1 lime
- ½ tablespoon cider vinegar or white wine vinegar
- 1 garlic clove, finely grated
- 1 teaspoon ground cumin
- 1 teaspoon ground cardamom
- ¼ teaspoon grains of paradise, crushed
- ½ teaspoon ajwain, crushed
- 7 tablespoons extra-virgin olive oil

**Directions**

1. Pierce each eggplant with the tip of a knife, you don't have to remove the tops and cut the tomatoes in half. Put them into a baking pan in a single layer.

2. Melt the butter in a saucepan and add the garlic. Cook over a low heat for a few minutes, then pour the butter all over the vegetables, turning them over. Season and sprinkle each tomato half with a little sugar if they aren't very sweet; if you have great tomatoes you won't need it.

3. Select Bake. Set temperature to 400°F (205°C) and set time to 40 minutes. Select Start to begin preheating.

4. Once preheated, slide the pan into the oven. Flip the eggplants halfway through the cooking time.

5. For the koch-kocha sauce, simply put everything into a food processor and whizz until smooth.

6. After 30 minutes, add the freekeh to the baking pan, pushing it down under the vegetables. Return to the oven for a final 10 minutes, or until the tomatoes are caramelized, the eggplants are tender right through, and the freekeh has become slightly sticky at the edges. Serve the dish with the sauce, a big bowl of plain yogurt, and good bread.

**Nutrition:** Calories 79 Carbs 7 g Protein 5 g Fat 3 g

# Cheesy Eggplant with Chili Smoked Almonds

Preparation time: 10 minutes

Cooking time: 45 minutes

Servings: 6

**Ingredients**

- 3¾ pounds (1.7 kg) globe eggplants
- 5 tablespoons extra-virgin olive oil
- 2 teaspoons harissa
- Sea salt flakes and freshly ground black pepper, to taste
- 2 garlic cloves, finely grated
- Juice of ½ lemon, or to taste
- 3½ ounces (99 g) goat curd or soft creamy goat cheese
- 1 tablespoon smoked almonds, roughly chopped (you want quite big bits)
- 2 red Fresno chilies, halved, seeded, and very thinly sliced
- Leaves from 1 rosemary sprig, chopped
- Warm flatbread or toasted sourdough bread, to serve

**Directions**

1. Put the eggplants in a baking pan and brush lightly with some of the olive oil. Pierce each a few times with the tines of a fork.
2. Select Bake. Set temperature to 400°F (205°C) and set time to 45 minutes. Select Start to begin preheating.
3. Once preheated, slide the pan into the oven.
4. When done, the eggplants will be completely soft and look a bit deflated.
5. Leave until cool enough to handle, then slit the skins and scoop the flesh out into a bowl. Chop the flesh. Mash, and add about 3½ tablespoons of the oil, the harissa, salt, pepper, garlic, and lemon juice to taste. Put this into a warmed serving bowl and scatter the goat cheese on top.
6. Heat the remaining extra-virgin olive oil in a frying pan and quickly fry the smoked almonds, chilies, and rosemary together. Pour this over the roast eggplants and serve with bread.

**Nutrition:** Calories 79 Carbs 7 g Protein 5 g Fat 3 g

# Butternut Squash with Goat Cheese

Preparation time: 5 minutes

Cooking time: 20 minutes

Servings: 2

## Ingredients

- 1 pound (454 g) butternut squash, cut into wedges
- 2 tablespoons olive oil
- 1 tablespoon dried rosemary
- Salt, to salt
- 1 cup crumbled goat cheese
- 1 tablespoon maple syrup

## Directions

1. Toss the squash wedges with the olive oil, rosemary, and salt in a large bowl until well coated.
2. Transfer the squash wedges to the perforated pan, spreading them out in as even a layer as possible.
3. Select Air Fry. Set temperature to 350°F (180°C) and set time to 20 minutes. Press Start to begin preheating.
4. Once preheated, place the pan into the oven.
5. After 10 minutes, remove from the oven and flip the squash. Return the pan to the oven and continue cooking for 10 minutes.

6. When cooking is complete, the squash should be golden brown. Remove the pan from the oven. Sprinkle the goat cheese on top and serve drizzled with the maple syrup.

**Nutrition:** Calories 79 Carbs 7 g Protein 5 g Fat 3 g

# Smoked Paprika Vegetable with Eggs

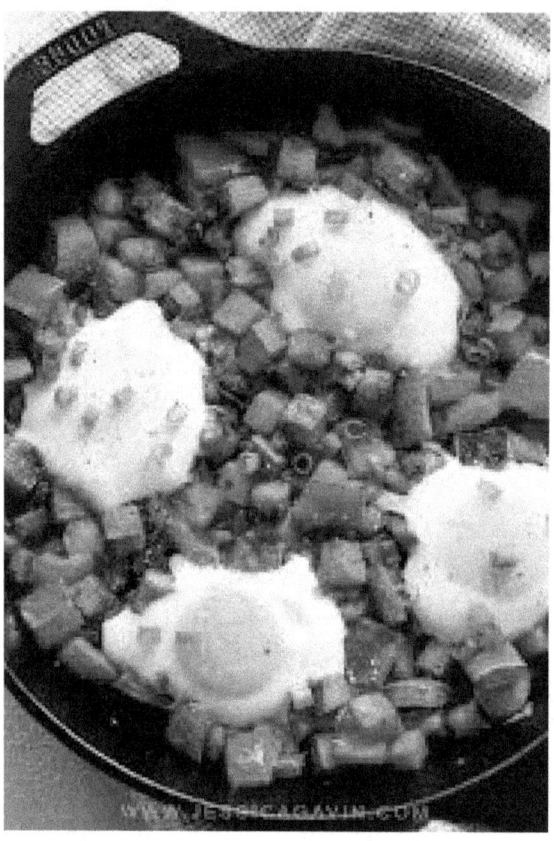

Preparation time: 15 minutes

Cooking time: 46 minutes

Servings: 4

**Ingredients**

- 4 zucchinis
- 1 pound (454 g) small waxy potatoes, scrubbed and quartered

- ⅔ pound (302 g) cherry tomatoes
- 12 scallions, trimmed
- 3 tablespoons extra-virgin olive oil
- Sea salt flakes and freshly ground black pepper, to taste
- Leaves from 3 thyme sprigs, plus 5 whole thyme sprigs
- ½ teaspoon crushed red pepper (optional)
- ¾ tablespoon smoked paprika, plus more to serve
- 4 garlic cloves, finely grated
- ½ pound (227 g) string beans, stem ends removed
- 6 to 8 extra-large eggs
- Greek yogurt, to serve (optional)

**Directions**

1. Trim the ends from the zucchini and cut them into ¼ in thick slices. Put all the vegetables except the string beans into a baking pan in a single layer. Add 2 tablespoons of the olive oil, the seasoning, thyme, crushed red pepper, smoked paprika, and garlic. Toss everything together.

2. Select Bake. Set temperature to 400°F (205°C) and set time to 46 minutes. Select Start to begin preheating.

3. Once preheated, slide the pan into the oven. Stir the vegetables over a couple of times.

4. After 30 minutes, toss the string beans with the remaining oil and scatter them on top of the other vegetables. Return to the oven for 8 minutes.

5. Break the eggs on top, season, and return the casserole or pan to the oven for a final 8 minutes or so. The eggs should be cooked.

6. Serve straight from the pan, sprinkling the eggs with a little more paprika, if you like. If you've made it very spicy and I often do a bowl of Greek yogurt on the side is good.

**Nutrition:** Calories 79 Carbs 7 g Protein 5 g Fat 3 g

# Double Cheese Roasted Asparagus

Preparation time: 5 minutes

Cooking time: 10 minutes

Servings: 4

**Ingredients**

- ⅔ pound (302 g) asparagus spears, of medium thickness
- Extra-virgin olive oil
- Sea salt flakes and freshly ground black pepper, to taste
- 4½ ounces (127 g) ricotta cheese (fresh rather than ultra-pasteurized, if possible)
- Pecorino cheese, or Parmesan cheese, shaved

**Directions**

1. Trim the woody ends from the asparagus spears, put them on a sheet pan with a slight lip, and drizzle with olive oil. Season with salt.
2. Select Bake. Set temperature to 400°F (205°C) and set time to 10 minutes. Select Start to begin preheating.
3. Once preheated, slide the pan into the oven.
4. When done, the asparagus spears will be tender.
5. Put the asparagus on a serving plate. Scatter the ricotta in nuggets over the top, followed by the shaved

pecorino or Parmesan cheese. Season with salt and pepper, pour on more olive oil, and serve immediately.

**Nutrition:** Calories 79 Carbs 7 g Protein 5 g Fat 3 g

# Chili Tomato with Herbs and Pistachios

Preparation time: 15 minutes

Cooking time: 30 minutes

Servings: 3

**Ingredients**

- 1⅔ pounds (756 g) plum tomatoes, halved lengthwise
- 4 tablespoons extra-virgin olive oil
- 3 teaspoons crushed red pepper
- 2 teaspoons fennel seeds
- Sea salt flakes and freshly ground black pepper, to taste
- 4 teaspoons clear honey
- 1 cup Greek yogurt, or more, depending on the size of your serving plate
- 1 cup crumbled Feta cheese
- 1 garlic clove, finely grated
- ⅓ cup dill, chopped, any thick stalks removed
- Scant 1 cup mint leaves
- 1 tablespoon chopped shelled unsalted pistachio nuts

**Directions**

1. Put all the tomatoes into a baking pan in which they can lie in a single layer; if they are too close to each other, they will steam instead of roasting. Spoon 3 tablespoons

of the oil over them, then turn them over with your hands so they get well coated. Leave them cut sides up.

2. Put the crushed red pepper and fennel seeds into a mortar and bash them. You won't break the fennel seeds down, but you'll crush them a bit. Sprinkle these over the tomatoes and season. Mix the honey with the remaining olive oil and spoon a little over each tomato.

3. Select Bake. Set temperature to 400°F (205°C) and set time to 30 minutes. Select Start to begin preheating.

4. Once preheated, slide the pan into the oven.

5. Keep an eye on them; you may find they need a little longer, but don't overcook them. They get to a point when they completely collapse and even though they're delicious at this stage, they've lost all their shape and you don't want that here.

6. Stir the yogurt, Feta, and garlic together and season. Put the yogurt mixture on a serving plate and pile the roast tomatoes on top. Sprinkle the herbs and pistachios all over the dish and serve.

**Nutrition:** Calories 79 Carbs 7 g Protein 5 g Fat 3 g

# Tomato and Black Olive Clafoutis

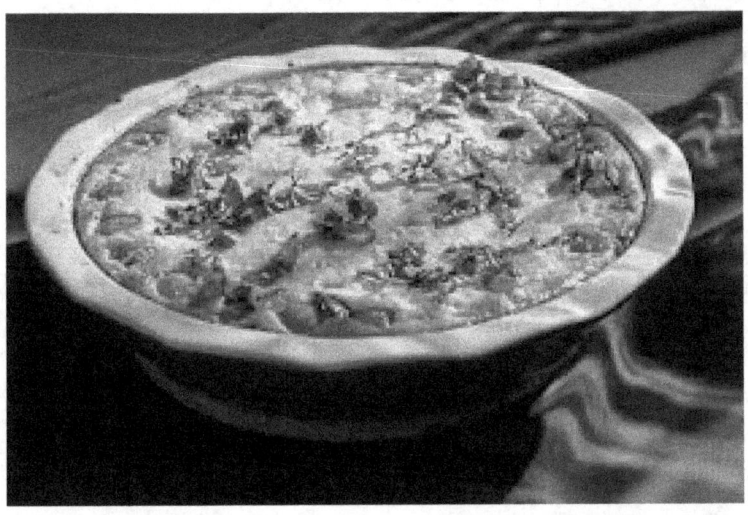

Preparation time: 15 minutes

Cooking time: 55 minutes

Servings: 6

**Ingredients**

- 1 pound (454 g) mixed cherry and plum tomatoes, halved or quartered, depending on size
- 1½ tablespoons extra-virgin olive oil
- Sea salt flakes and freshly ground black pepper, to taste
- 4 large eggs, plus
- 2 large egg yolks
- ⅓ cup all-purpose flour
- Scant 1 cup milk

- 1¼ cups heavy cream
- Generous ½ cup finely grated Parmesan cheese
- 1 garlic clove, finely grated
- 2 tablespoons chopped pitted black olives
- 7 ounces (198 g) soft goat cheese, crumbled
- ⅓ cup basil leaves, torn

## Directions

1. Put the tomatoes into a gratin dish with the olive oil and season them. Turn them over so the surfaces are all coated in a little oil.

2. Select Bake. Set temperature to 400°F (205°C) and set time to 25 minutes. Select Start to begin preheating.

3. Once preheated, slide the dish into the oven.

4. When done, the tomatoes will be soft and slightly shrunken. Take out of the oven and leave to sit on a work surface.

5. Reduce the oven temperature to 375°F (190°C).

6. Put the eggs, egg yolks, flour, milk, and cream into a food processor, season well, and whizz. Stir in the Parmesan and garlic.

7. Scatter the olives over the tomatoes and crumble on the goat cheese.

8. Pour the batter over the tomatoes, olives, and cheese and bake for 30 minutes, until the custard is puffed, golden, and just set in the middle. Leave it for 5

minutes to settle: it will sink a little once it has sat for a while. Scatter over the basil and serve.

**Nutrition:** Calories 79 Carbs 7 g Protein 5 g Fat 3 g

# SNACKS

## Chicken with Herbs and Cream

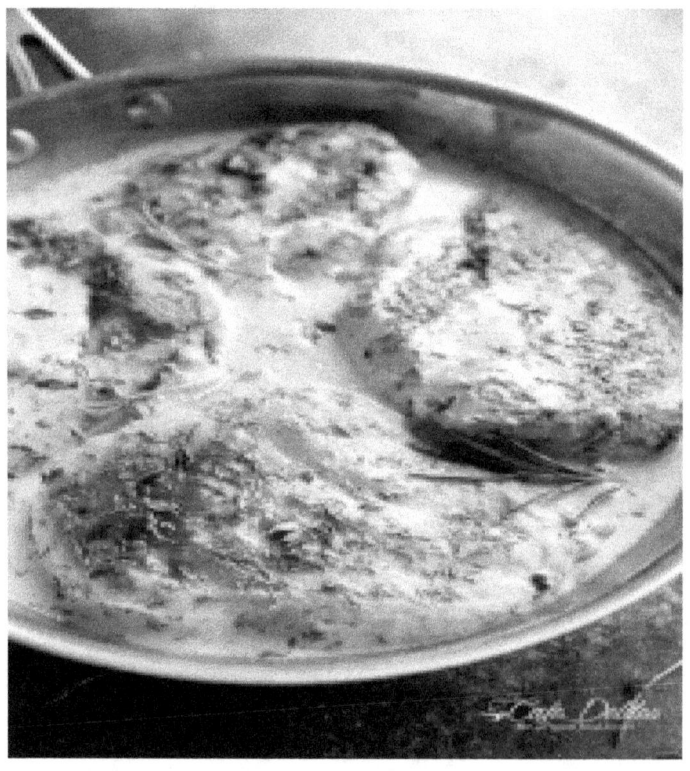

Preparation Time: 5 to 10 Minutes

Cooking Time: 15 Minutes

Servings: 4

**Ingredients:**

- 4 ounces garlic and herb cream cheese
- Salt and pepper to taste
- 2 teaspoons dried Italian seasoning
- Olive oil as needed
- 2 chicken breast fillets

**Directions:**

1. Take the chicken and brush them with oil
2. Season them with salt, pepper, and Italian seasoning
3. Top them with garlic and herb cream cheese
4. Roll up the chicken carefully
5. Transfer them to the Air Crisping basket
6. Place the basket inside the appliance
7. AIR CRISP for 7 minutes per side, at 370 degrees F
8. Serve and enjoy!

**Nutrition:** Calories: 750, Fat: 42 g, Saturated Fat: 10 g, Carbohydrates: 18 g, Fiber: 3 g, Sodium: 846 mg, Protein: 73 g

# Meaty Bratwursts

Preparation Time: 5 to 10 Minutes

Cooking Time: 12 Minutes

Servings: 4

**Ingredients:**

- 1 pack bratwursts

**Directions:**

1. Preheat your Ninja Foodi Smart XL Grill in AIR CRISP mode for 5 minutes at 350 degrees F
2. Add bratwurst to the Cooking basket
3. Cook for 10 minutes, making sure to flip once
4. Enjoy!

**Nutrition:** Calories: 739 Fat: 57 g, Saturated Fat: 20 g Carbohydrates: 13 g Fiber: 3 g Sodium: 2641 mg Protein: 37 g

# Delicious Taco Cups

Preparation Time: 5 to 10 Minutes

Cooking Time: 10 Minutes

Servings: 4

**Ingredients:**

- 1 cup cheddar cheese, shredded
- 2 tablespoons taco seasoning
- ½ cup tomatoes, chopped
- 1-pound ground beef, cooked
- 12 wonton wrappers

**Directions:**

1. Press wrappers firmly onto the muffin pan
2. Transfer the pan inside your Ninja Foodi Smart XL Grill
3. Air Fry on AIR CRISP mode for 5 minutes at 400 degrees F
4. Top with ground beef and tomatoes,
5. Sprinkle taco seasoning, cheese
6. Air Fry for 5 minutes more
7. Enjoy!

**Nutrition:** Calories: 431, Fat: 21 g, Saturated Fat: 7 g, Carbohydrates: 30 g, Fiber: 5 g, Sodium: 604 mg, Protein: 31 g

# Mustard and Veggie

Preparation Time: 5 to 10 Minutes

Cooking Time: 30 to 40 Minutes

Servings: 4

**Ingredients:**

- Vinaigrette
- ½ cup olive oil
- ½ cup avocado oil
- ¼ teaspoon pepper
- 1 teaspoon salt
- 2 tablespoons honey
- ½ cup red wine vinegar
- 2 tablespoons Dijon vinegar
- Veggies
- 4 zucchinis, halved
- 4 sweet onion, quartered
- 4 red pepper, seeded and halved
- 2 bunch green onions, trimmed
- 4 yellow squash, cut in half

**Directions:**

1. Take a small bowl and whisk in mustard, honey, vinegar, salt, and pepper. Add oil and mix well

2. Set your Ninja Foodi Smart XL Grill to GRILL mode and MED setting, set timer to 10 minutes

3. Transfer onion quarter to Grill Grate, cook for 5 minutes

4. Flip and cook for 5 minutes more

5. Grill remaining veggies in the same way, giving 7 minutes per side for zucchini and 1 minute for green onions

6. Serve with mustard vinaigrette on top

7. Enjoy!

**Nutrition:** Calories: 327, Fat: 5 g, Saturated Fat: 0.5 g, Carbohydrates:328 g, Fiber: 2 g, Sodium: 524 mg, Protein: 8 g

# Season Garlic Carrots

Preparation Time: 5 to 10 Minutes

Cooking Time: 10 Minutes

Servings: 4

**Ingredients:**

- Salt and pepper to taste
- 2 teaspoons garlic powder
- 2 tablespoons olive oil
- 1-pound carrots, diced

**Directions:**

1. Take a bowl and toss the carrot cubes generously in oil
2. Season the cube further with salt, pepper, and garlic powder
3. Make sure that they are coated evenly
4. Spread the carrots in the Air Crisp Basket
5. Set your Ninja Foodi Smart XL Grill to 390 degrees F in AIR CRISP mode and set the timer to 30 minutes
6. Cook for 10 minutes, making sure to stir once
7. Serve and enjoy!

**Nutrition:** Calories: 183, Fat: 11 g, Saturated Fat: 5 g, Carbohydrates: 21 g, Fiber: 1 g, Sodium: 440 mg, Protein: 2 g

# Sausage Patties

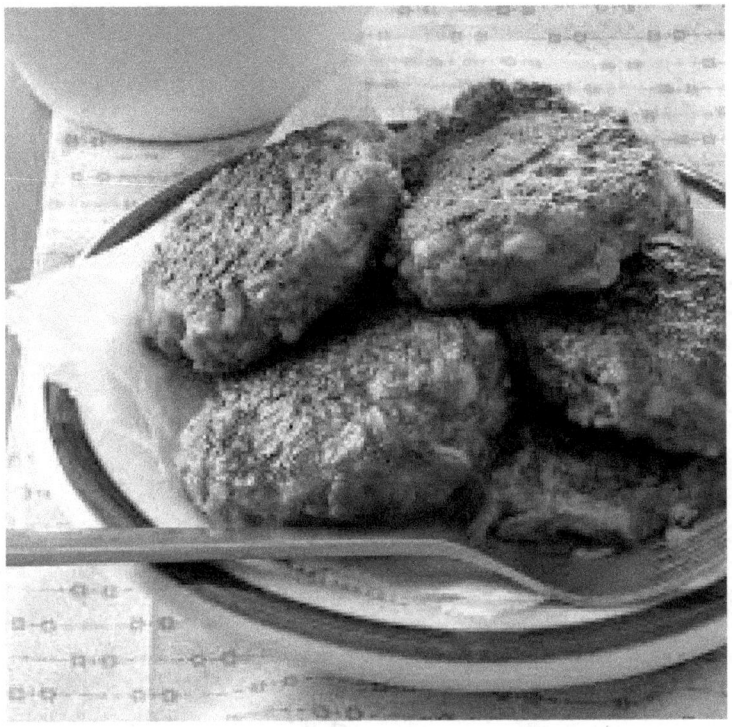

Preparation Time: 5 to 10 Minutes

Cooking Time: 10 Minutes

Servings: 2

**Ingredients:**

- 1 pack sausage patties

**Directions:**

1. Transfer sausages to the Air Fryer cooking basket
2. Select the Air Crisp Mode and set the temperature to 400 degrees F
3. Cook for 5 minutes per side
4. Serve and enjoy once done!

**Nutrition:** Calories: 228 Fat: 13 g Saturated Fat: 5 g Carbohydrates: 5 g Fiber: 2 g Sodium: 145 mg Protein: 21 g

# Cute Mozzarella Bites

Preparation Time: 5 to 10 Minutes

Cooking Time: 8 Minutes

Servings: 12

**Ingredients:**

- 1 cup breadcrumbs
- ¼ cup butter, melted
- 12 mozzarella strips

**Directions:**

1. Dip the mozzarella strips in butter
2. Dredge them with breadcrumbs
3. Add mozzarella strips to your Ninja Foodi Smart XL Grill Crisping basket
4. Cook at 320 degrees F for 8 minutes on AIR CRISP mode
5. Cook for 8 minutes, making sure to flip once
6. Serve and enjoy!

**Nutrition:** Calories: 206, Fat: 12 g, Saturated Fat: 5 g, Carbohydrates: 16 g, Fiber: 5 g, Sodium: 284 mg, Protein: 10 g

# Simple Garlic Bread

Preparation Time: 5 to 10 Minutes

Cooking Time: 5 Minutes

Servings: 4

**Ingredients:**

- Salt to taste
- 1 Italian loaf of bread
- 1 tablespoon fresh parsley, chopped
- ½ cup butter, melted
- 4 garlic cloves, chopped

**Directions:**

1. Take a bowl and add parsley, butter, and garlic
2. Spread the mixture on the bread slices
3. Transfer the bread inside the Ninja Foodi Smart XL Grill cooking basket
4. Cook at 400 degrees F for 3 minutes on AIR CRISP mode
5. Serve and enjoy once done

**Nutrition:** Calories: 155, Fat: 7 g, Saturated Fat: 2 g, Carbohydrates: 20 g, Fiber: 3 g, Sodium: 227 mg, Protein: 28 g

# Particularly Crispy Tomatoes

Preparation Time: 5 to 10 Minutes

Cooking Time: 5 Minutes

Servings: 4

**Ingredients:**

- Bread crumbs as needed
- ½ cup buttermilk
- ¼ cup almond flour
- Salt and pepper to taste
- ¼ tablespoon Creole seasoning
- 1 green tomato

**Directions:**

1. Preheat Ninja Foodi Smart XL Grill by pressing the "AIR CRISP" option and setting it to "400 Degrees F" and timer to 5 minutes
2. let it preheat until you hear a beep
3. Add flour to your plate and take another plate and add buttermilk
4. Cut tomatoes and season with salt and pepper
5. Make a mix of creole seasoning and crumbs
6. Take tomato slice and cover with flour, place in buttermilk and then into crumbs
7. Repeat with all tomatoes

8. Cook the tomato slices for 5 minutes

9. Serve with basil and enjoy!

**Nutrition:** Calories: 200, Fat: 12 g, Saturated Fat: 4 g, Carbohydrates: 11 g, Fiber: 2 g, Sodium: 1203 mg, Protein: 3 g

# Healthy Blueberry Muffins

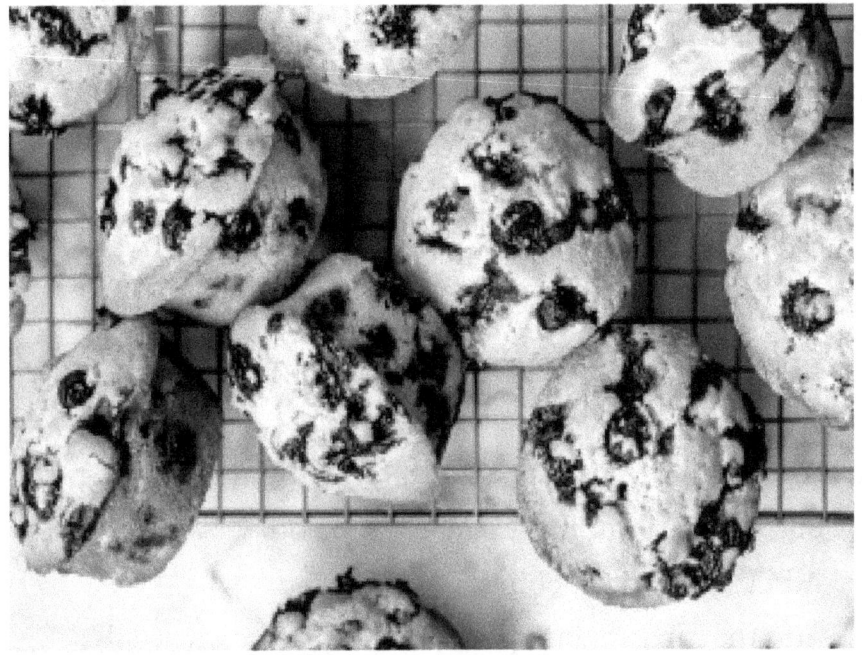

Preparation Time: 10 Minutes

Cooking Time: 10 Minutes

Servings: 8 to 10

**Ingredients:**

- 2 teaspoons vanilla extract
- 1 cup blueberries
- ½ teaspoon salt
- 1 cup yogurt
- 1 ½ cups cake flour

- ½ cup sugar
- 2 teaspoons baking powder
- 1/3 cup vegetable oil
- 1 egg

**Directions:**

1. Place your air fryer on a flat kitchen surface; plug it and turn it on. Set temperature to 355 degrees F and let it preheat for 4-5 minutes.
2. Take 10 muffin molds and gently coat them using a cooking oil or spray.
3. In a bowl of medium size, thoroughly mix the flour, sugar, baking powder and salt.
4. In a bowl of medium size, thoroughly mix the yogurt, oil, egg and vanilla extract. Mix both bowl mixtures. Add the chocolate chips.
5. Add the mixture into prepared muffin molds evenly.
6. Add the molds in the basket. Push the air-frying basket in the air fryer. Cook for 10 minutes.
7. Slide out the basket; serve warm!

**Nutrition:** Calories - 214 Fat – 8g Carbohydrates – 32g Fiber – 1g Protein – 4g

# DESSERTS

## Novella Banana Pastries

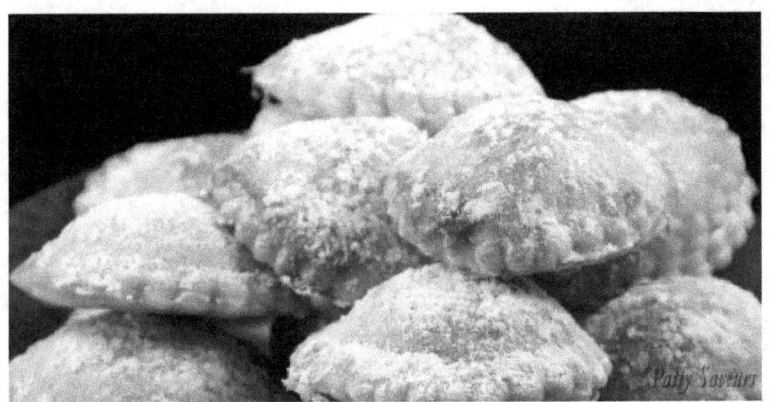

Preparation Time: 15 minutes

Cooking Time: 12 minutes

Servings: 4

**Ingredients:**

- One puff pastry sheet
- ½ cup Novella
- Two bananas, peeled and sliced

**Directions**

1. Cut the pastry sheet into four equal-sized squares.
2. Spread the Novella on each square of pastry evenly.
3. Divide the banana slices over Novella.
4. Fold each square into a triangle, and with wet fingers, slightly press the edges.
5. Then with a fork, press the edges firmly.
6. Press "Power Button" of Air Fry Oven and turn the dial to select the "Air Fry" mode.
7. Set the cooking time to 12 minutes.
8. Now push the Temp button and rotate the dial to set the temperature at 375 degrees F.
9. Press the "Start/Pause" button to start.
10. When the unit beeps it means that it is preheated, open the lid.
11. Arrange the pastries in a greased "Air Fry Basket" and insert them in the oven.
12. Serve warm.

**Nutrition:** Calories 221 Total Fat 10 g Sodium 103 mg Total Carbs 31.6 g  Fiber 2.6 g Protein 3.4 g

# Lemon Mousse

Preparation Time: 15 minutes
Cooking Time: 12 minutes
Servings: 2
**Ingredients:**

- 4 oz. cream cheese softened
- ½ cup heavy cream
- 2 tbsp. fresh lemon juice
- 4-6 drops liquid stevia
- Two pinches salt

**Directions**

1. In a bowl, add all the ingredients and mix until well combined.
2. Transfer the mixture into two ramekins.
3. Press "Power Button" of Air Fry Oven and turn the dial to select the "Air Bake" mode.
4. Set the cooking time to 12 minutes.
5. Now push the Temp button and rotate the dial to set the temperature at 350 degrees F.
6. Press the "Start/Pause" button to start.
7. When the unit beeps it means that it is preheated, open the lid.
8. Arrange the ramekins over the "Wire Rack" and insert them in the oven.
9. Place the ramekins onto a wire rack to cool.
10. Refrigerate for at least 3 hours before serving.

**Nutrition:** Calories 305 Total Fat 31 g Sodium 337 mg Total Carbs 2.7 g  Fiber 0.1 g Protein 5 g

# Chocolate Pudding

Preparation Time: 20 minutes

Cooking Time: 12 minutes

Servings: 4

**Ingredients:**

- ½ cup butter
- 2/3 cup dark chocolate, chopped
- ¼ cup caster sugar
- 2 medium eggs
- 2 tsp. fresh orange rind, finely grated
- ¼ cup fresh orange juice
- 2 tbsp. self-rising flour

**Directions**

1. In a microwave-safe bowl, add the butter and chocolate and microwave on high heat for about 2 minutes or until melted completely, stirring after every 30 seconds.
2. Remove from the microwave and stir the mixture until smooth.
3. Add the sugar and eggs and whisk until frothy.
4. Add the orange rind and juice, followed by flour and mix until well combined.
5. Divide mixture into four greased ramekins about ¾ full.

6. Press "Power Button" of Air Fry Oven and turn the dial to select the "Air Fry" mode.

7. Set the cooking time to 12 minutes.

8. Now push the Temp button and rotate the dial to set the temperature at 355 degrees F.

9. Press the "Start/Pause" button to start.

10. When the unit beeps it means that it is preheated, open the lid.

11. Arrange the ramekins in "Air Fry Basket" and insert them in the oven.

12. Place the ramekins set aside to cool completely before serving.

**Nutrition:** Calories 454 Total Fat 33.6 g Sodium 217 mg Total Carbs 34.2 g Fiber 1.2 g Protein 5.7 g

# Chocolate Soufflé

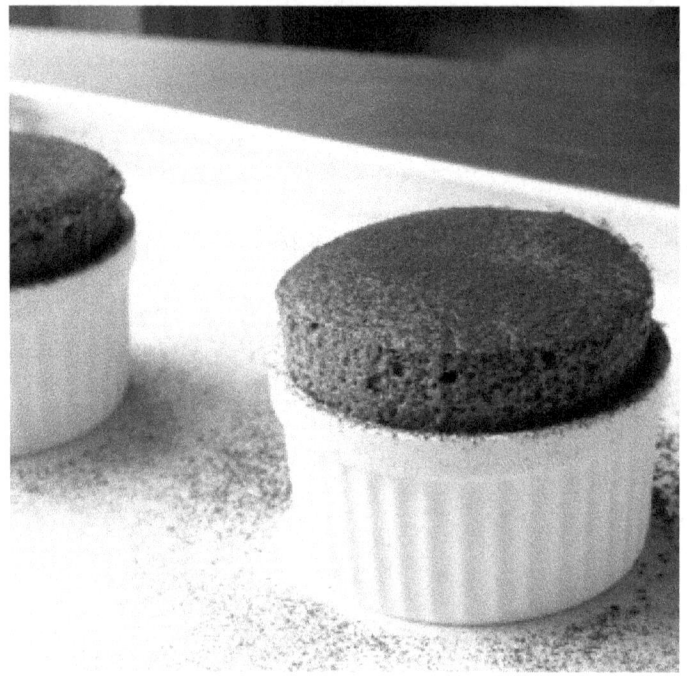

Preparation Time: 15 minutes

Cooking Time: 16 minutes

Servings: 2

## Ingredients:

- 3 oz. semi-sweet chocolate, chopped
- ¼ cup butter
- Two eggs, yolks and whites separated
- 3 tbsp. sugar
- ½ tsp. pure vanilla extract

- 2 tbsp. all-purpose flour
- 1 tsp. powdered sugar plus extra for dusting

**Directions**

1. In a microwave-safe bowl, place the butter and chocolate. Microwave on high heat for about 2 minutes or until melted completely, stirring after every 30 seconds.
2. Remove from the microwave and stir the mixture until smooth.
3. In another bowl, add the egg yolks and whisk well.
4. Add the sugar and vanilla extract and whisk well.
5. Add the chocolate mixture and mix until well combined.
6. Add the flour and mix well.
7. In a clean glass bowl, add the egg whites and whisk until soft peaks form.
8. Fold the whipped egg whites in 3 portions into the chocolate mixture.
9. Grease 2 ramekins and sprinkle each with a pinch of sugar.
10. Place mixture into the prepared ramekins, and with the back of a spoon, smooth the top surface.
11. Press "Power Button" of Air Fry Oven and turn the dial to select the "Air Fry" mode.
12. Set the cooking time to 14 minutes.
13. Now push the Temp button and rotate the dial to set the temperature at 330 degrees F.

14. Press the "Start/Pause" button to start.

15. When the unit beeps it means that it is preheated, open the lid.

16. Arrange the ramekins in "Air Fry Basket" and insert them in the oven.

17. Place the ramekins onto a wire rack to cool slightly.

18. Sprinkle with the powdered sugar and serve warm.

**Nutrition:** Calories 591 Total Fat 38.7 g Sodium 225 mg Total Carbs 52.6 g  Fiber 0.2 g Protein 9.4 g

# Fudge Brownies

Preparation Time: 15 minutes

Cooking Time: 20 minutes

Servings: 8

**Ingredients:**

- 1 cup sugar
- ½ cup butter, melted
- ½ cup flour
- 1/3 cup cocoa powder
- 1 tsp. baking powder
- 2 eggs
- 1 tsp. vanilla extract

**Directions**

1. Grease a baking pan.
2. In a large bowl, add the sugar and butter and whisk until light and fluffy.
3. Add the remaining ingredients and mix until well combined.
4. Place mixture into the prepared pan, and with the back of the spatula, smooth the top surface.
5. Press "Power Button" of Air Fry Oven and turn the dial to select the "Air Fry" mode.
6. Set the cooking time to 20 minutes.

7. Now push the Temp button and rotate the dial to set the temperature at 350 degrees F.

8. Press the "Start/Pause" button to start.

9. When the unit beeps it means that it is preheated, open the lid.

10. Arrange the pan in "Air Fry Basket" and insert it in the oven.

11. Place the baking pan onto a wire rack to cool completely.

12. Cut into eight equal-sized squares and serve.

**Nutrition:** Calories 250 Total Fat 13.2 g Sodium 99 mg Total Carbs 33.4 g  Fiber 1.3 g Protein 3 g

# Walnut Brownies

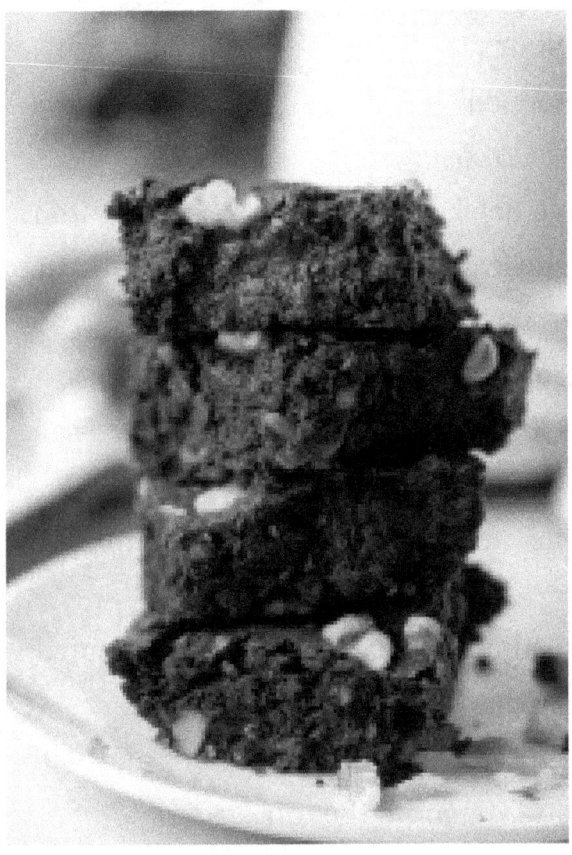

Preparation Time: 15 minutes

Cooking Time: 22 minutes

Servings: 4

**Ingredients:**

- ½ cup chocolate, roughly chopped
- 1/3 cup butter

- 5 tbsp. sugar
- 1 egg, beaten
- 1 tsp. vanilla extract
- Pinch of salt
- 5 tbsp. self-rising flour
- ¼ cup walnuts, chopped

**Directions**

1. In a microwave-safe bowl, add the chocolate and butter. Microwave on high heat for about 2 minutes, stirring after every 30 seconds.
2. Remove from microwave and set aside to cool.
3. In another bowl, add the sugar, egg, vanilla extract, salt, and whisk until creamy and light.
4. Add the chocolate mixture and whisk until well combined.
5. Add the flour and walnuts and mix until well combined.
6. Line a baking pan with a greased parchment paper.
7. Place mixture evenly into the prepared pan, and with the back of the spatula, smooth the top surface.
8. Press "Power Button" of Air Fry Oven and turn the dial to select the "Air Fry" mode.
9. Set the cooking time to 20 minutes.
10. Now push the Temp button and rotate the dial to set the temperature at 355 degrees F.
11. Press the "Start/Pause" button to start.

12. When the unit beeps it means that it is preheated, open the lid.

13. Arrange the pan in "Air Fry Basket" and insert it in the oven.

14. Place the baking pan onto a wire rack to cool completely.

15. Cut into four equal-sized squares and serve.

**Nutrition:** Calories 407 Total Fat 27.4g Sodium 180 mg Total Carbs 35.9 g  Fiber 1.5 g Protein 6 g

# Nutella Banana Muffins

Preparation Time: 15 minutes

Cooking Time: 25 minutes

Servings: 12

**Ingredients:**

- 1 2/3 cups plain flour
- 1 tsp. baking soda
- 1 tsp. baking powder
- 1 tsp. ground cinnamon
- ¼ tsp. salt
- Four ripe bananas, peeled and mashed
- Two eggs
- ½ cup brown sugar
- 1 tsp. vanilla essence
- 3 tbsp. milk
- 1 tbsp. Nutella
- ¼ cup walnuts

**Directions**

1. Grease 12 muffin molds. Set aside.
2. In a large bowl, sift together the flour, baking soda, baking powder, cinnamon, and salt.
3. In another bowl, mix the remaining ingredients except for walnuts.

4. Add the banana mixture into the flour mixture and mix until just combined.
5. Fold in the walnuts.
6. Place the mixture into the prepared muffin molds.
7. Press "Power Button" of Air Fry Oven and turn the dial to select the "Air Fry" mode.
8. Seethe cooking time to 25 minutes.
9. Now push the Temp button and rotate the dial to set the temperature at 250 degrees F.
10. Press the "Start/Pause" button to start.
11. When the unit beeps it means that it is preheated, open the lid.
12. Arrange the muffin molds in "Air Fry Basket" and insert them in the oven.
13. Place the muffin molds onto a wire rack to cool for about 10 minutes.
14. Carefully invert the muffins onto the wire rack to completely cool before serving.

**Nutrition:** Calories 227 Total Fat 6.6 g Sodium 221 mg Total Carbs 38.1 g Fiber 2.4 g Protein 5.2 g

# Blueberry Muffins

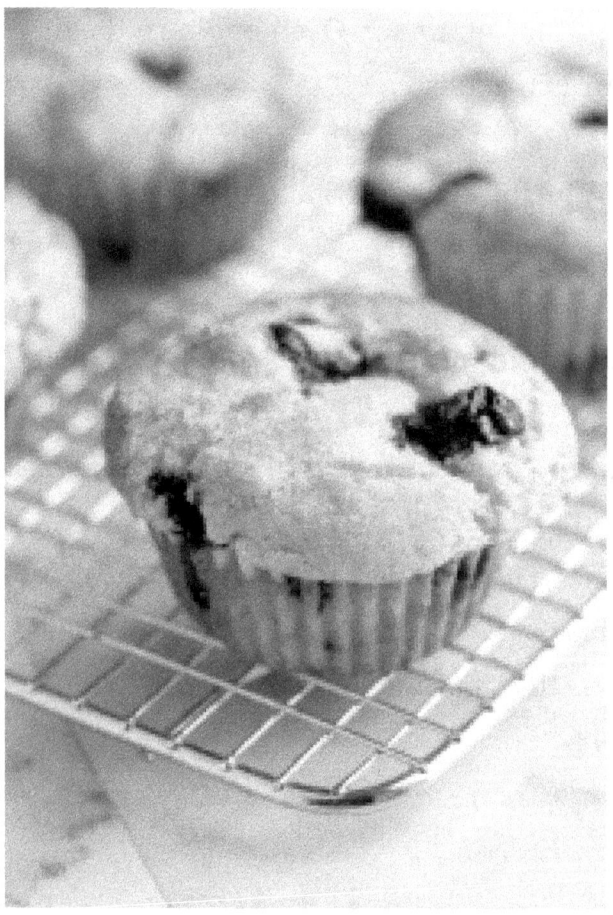

Preparation Time: 15 minutes

Cooking Time: 12 minutes

Servings: 12

**Ingredients:**

- 2 cups plus 2 tbsp. self-rising flour

- 5 tbsp. white sugar
- ½ cup milk
- 2 oz. butter, melted
- 2 eggs
- 2 tsp. fresh orange zest, finely grated
- 2 tbsp. fresh orange juice
- ½ tsp. vanilla extract
- ½ cup fresh blueberries

**Directions**

1. Grease 12 muffin molds. Set aside.
2. In a bowl, mix the flour and white sugar.
3. In another large bowl, mix well the remaining ingredients except for blueberries.
4. Add the flour mixture and mix until just combined.
5. Fold in the blueberries.
6. Place the mixture into the prepared muffin molds.
7. Press "Power Button" of Air Fry Oven and turn the dial to select the "Air Fry" mode.
8. Set the cooking time to 12 minutes.
9. Now push the Temp button and rotate the dial to set the temperature at 355 degrees F.
10. Press the "Start/Pause" button to start.
11. When the unit beeps it means that it is preheated, open the lid.
12. Arrange the muffin molds in "Air Fry Basket" and insert them in the oven.

13. Place the muffin molds onto a wire rack to cool for about 10 minutes.

14. Carefully invert the muffins onto the wire rack to completely cool before serving.

**Nutrition:** Calories 149 Total Fat 5 g Sodium 43 mg Total Carbs 22.7 g  Fiber 0.8 g Protein 3.5 g

# Cranberry Muffins

Preparation Time: 15 minutes

Cooking Time: 15 minutes

Servings: 8

**Ingredients:**

- ¼ cup unsweetened almond milk
- Two large eggs
- ½ tsp. vanilla extract
- 1½ cups almond flour
- ¼ cup Erythritol
- 1 tsp. baking powder
- ¼ tsp. ground cinnamon
- 1/8 tsp. salt
- ½ cup fresh cranberries
- ¼ cup walnuts, chopped

**Directions**

1. In a blender, add the almond milk, eggs, vanilla extract and pulse for about 20-30 seconds.
2. Add the almond flour, Erythritol, baking powder, cinnamon, salt, and pulse for about 30-45 seconds until well blended.
3. Transfer the mixture into a bowl.
4. Gently fold in half of the cranberries and walnuts.

5. Place the mixture into eight silicone muffin cups and top each with remaining cranberries.
6. Press "Power Button" of Air Fry Oven and turn the dial to select the "Air Fry" mode.
7. Set the cooking time to 15 minutes.
8. Now push the Temp button and rotate the dial to set the temperature at 325 degrees F.
9. Press the "Start/Pause" button to start.
10. When the unit beeps it means that it is preheated, open the lid.
11. Arrange the muffin cups in "Air Fry Basket" and insert them in the oven.
12. Place the muffin molds onto a wire rack to cool for about 10 minutes.
13. Carefully invert the muffins onto the wire rack to completely cool before serving.

**Nutrition:** Calories 175 Fat 13.6 g Sodium 66 mg Total Carbs 6.1 g  Fiber 2.9 g Protein 7 g

# Brownie Muffins

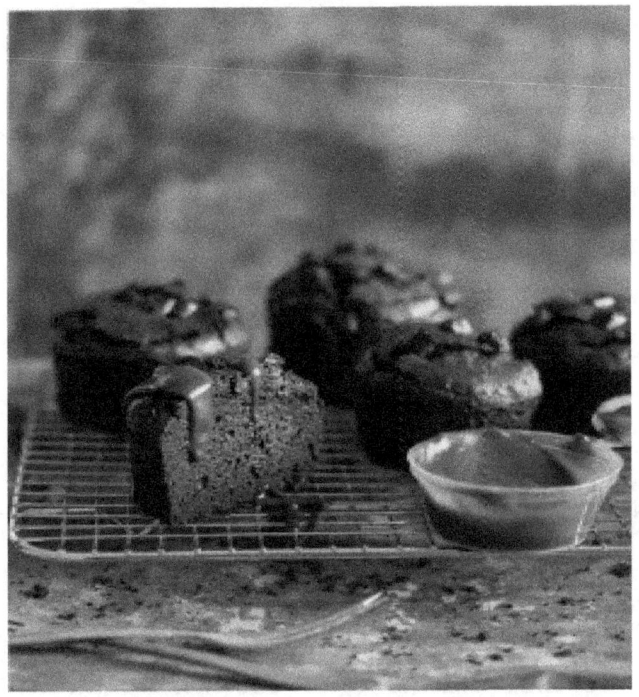

Preparation Time: 10 minutes

Cooking Time: 10 minutes

Servings: 12

## Ingredients:

- One package Betty Crocker fudges brownie mix
- ¼ cup walnuts, chopped
- One egg
- 1/3 cup vegetable oil
- 2 tsp. water

## Directions

1. Grease 12 muffin molds. Set aside.
2. In a bowl, mix all the ingredients.
3. Place the mixture into the prepared muffin molds.
4. Press "Power Button" of Air Fry Oven and turn the dial to select the "Air Fry" mode.
5. Set the cooking time to 10 minutes.
6. Now push the Temp button and rotate the dial to set the temperature at 300 degrees F.
7. Press the "Start/Pause" button to start.
8. When the unit beeps it means that it is preheated, open the lid.
9. Arrange the muffin molds in "Air Fry Basket" and insert them in the oven.
10. Place the muffin molds onto a wire rack to cool for about 10 minutes.
11. Carefully invert the muffins onto the wire rack to completely cool before serving.

**Nutrition:** Calories 168 Total Fat 8.9 g Sodium 89 mg Total Carbs 20.8 g Fiber 1.1 gProtein 2 g

# CONCLUSION

Below are some frequently asked questions and tips about air fryer that will help you.

Does Air Fryer need time to heat up?

No, the unit has a smart heating feature that heats up the unit to the set temperature before the times start to count down. The smart feature takes effect on all preset settings except dehydrate, bagel, and toast.

Is Air Fryer healthy?

Yes, Air Fryer makes an alternative to your favorite unhealthy fried food using air and not oil. Foods cooked with this unit have about 70% fewer calories compared to the deep-fried food.

How much energy does Air Fryer consume?

It consumes far less power than other many cooking appliances which saves on energy and money.

Do I need to use oil?

No, you don't need oil to get your food crispy. You may, however, spray a little oil to add more flavor.

Can I choose my own temperature and time?

Yes, you may manually set the preferred temperature and time as recommended on the recipe instead of using the one-touch preset functions.

Can I check my food during the cooking process?

Yes, you just need to press the Start/Pause button to pause the cooking process then open the door. Close the door and press the same button to resume cooking.

Tips

- Cut food into small pieces as it will require less time to cook.
- Flipping the food halfway through the cooking process ensures even cooked food.
- Mist a little oil on foodies. potatoes or meat for a crispier result.
- Use pre-made dough instead of homemade dough for quick and easy snacks.
- You can use a baking dish or a baking tin by placing it on the rack to cook quiches and cakes.

Cleaning and Maintenance

- You should clean the Air Fryer after every single use.
- Remove the power cord from the power sauce and ensure the gadget has completely cooled.

- Use a damp cloth with some mild detergent to wipe the outside.

- Gently scrub the door with a damp cloth and warm soapy water. The unit should never be soaked in water.

- Remove any food residue with a nonabrasive brush if it's necessary.

- Clean the inside with a nonabrasive sponge, hot water, and some mild detergent. Avoid scrubbing the heating elements since they are fragile and may break. Rinse the inside with a clean damp cloth.

- The accessories should be soaked in warm, soapy water and hand-washed so that the food residue can be easily removed.

- Make sure that the unit and its components are clean and dry before storing them in a clean and dry place.

Tips for Cooking Success

- Make sure that you follow the initial steps required before using the appliance.

- Foods that are smaller in size will require less cooking time. If you want to cut down on cooking time, cutting food into similar sizes will guarantee faster and even cooking.

- Spraying, misting, or lightly coating, food with oil before cooking will create a crispier texture. Be careful not to put too much, or it will turn soggy instead.

- Make sure that you flip or stir the food halfway through the cooking time to get even cooking.

- Snack or pastry recipes intended for conventional ovens may also be made in the air fryer oven.

- Avoid overcrowding the food. Leave some space in between, especially when cooking food with coating or batter, to let the hot air circulate and cook the food on all sides.

- For recipes that require high temperatures, it is better to use oils that have a high smoking point or that can withstand high temperatures. Avocado, peanut, and grapeseed oils are excellent examples of this. Olive oil has a low smoke point. If you must use olive oil, use extra light olive oil as it has a higher smoke point and will not dry up the food before it cooks.

- Do not place cooking trays or pans directly on the bottom heating elements as this will prevent the hot air to properly circulate and cook food.

- Crumbs and drippings like oil and grease can create smoke and burn. To prevent this, put a baking tray lined with foil and parchment paper and place it below the crisper tray or baking pan.

•

CPSIA information can be obtained
at www.ICGtesting.com
Printed in the USA
LVHW011445130421
684339LV00002B/162